Dr Barbara Cayenne Pepper Manual

The Complete Guide on Barbara Oneill Healing Recipes and Natural Remedies for Enhancing Immunity and Restore Health

ISBN 978-1-300-89159-8
Josef Panker
Copyright@2024

TABLE OF CONTENT

CHAPTER 1

INTRODUCTION

Cayenne pepper, a striking red chili pepper, is celebrated for its potent health advantages and diverse medicinal applications. This has been cherished for ages, serving not just as a flavorful addition to dishes but also as an essential natural treatment in various traditional healing practices worldwide. This powerful pepper derives a significant portion of its therapeutic benefits from its active compound, capsaicin, which imparts cayenne its distinctive heat. Capsaicin is celebrated for its remarkable properties in reducing inflammation, alleviating pain, and enhancing immune function. Furthermore, cayenne boasts a wealth of vitamins, particularly Vitamin A, which is crucial for immune system support, and Vitamin C, a potent antioxidant recognized for its ability to combat free radicals, lessen oxidative stress, and bolster immune strength.

Another distinctive characteristic of cayenne pepper is its thermogenic effect on the body. Incorporating cayenne pepper into your diet can lead to a temporary rise in body temperature, promoting enhanced blood circulation and supporting the detoxification process. Enhanced circulation facilitates the effective delivery of oxygen and nutrients to cells, which is vital for immune function and overall well-being. Moreover, the thermogenic qualities of cayenne contribute to enhancing metabolism, facilitating weight loss and diminishing inflammation. The digestive advantages are noteworthy, as cayenne has the ability to enhance the production of gastric juices, leading to improved digestion and helping to prevent issues like bloating and constipation. Cayenne pepper, with its unique properties, emerges as a remarkable natural remedy, adept at tackling a range of health concerns, including digestive issues, inflammation, and weakened immunity.

This guide delves into the ways cayenne pepper can be utilized to boost immunity and restore health, leveraging its natural attributes to ease different ailments and foster a comprehensive approach to wellness.

Exploring Barbara O'Neill's Method for Promoting Wellness and Strengthening Immunity

Barbara O'Neill is a highly regarded proponent of natural health, recognized for her thorough methodology that emphasizes a holistic treatment of the body instead of merely targeting isolated symptoms. Her philosophy revolves around the belief that the human body functions as an interconnected system, flourishing when its needs are fulfilled through wholesome, nutrient-dense foods, botanical remedies, and mindful lifestyle choices. O'Neill highlights the significance of incorporating natural solutions, modifying dietary habits, and making lifestyle alterations to enhance immune function and promote overall well-being. This approach resonates deeply with her conviction in the importance of preventive care—emphasizing practices that bolster immunity and diminish the risk of illness.

O'Neill's methodology emphasizes the essential importance of natural foods and botanicals in supporting a harmonious immune system. She promotes the use of natural remedies such as cayenne pepper, which are accessible, cost-effective, and potent in their healing properties. By harnessing the properties of cayenne, she illustrates how straightforward yet powerful natural solutions can act as primary safeguards against illness. At the heart of O'Neill's teachings lies the principle of "food as medicine," with cayenne pepper serving as a prime example of how intentional dietary selections can transform into potent allies in fostering health and vitality. In contrast to synthetic medications that frequently carry various side effects, cayenne and other natural remedies interact seamlessly with the body, promoting a natural healing process.

Alongside dietary choices, Barbara O'Neill emphasizes the significance of lifestyle practices like exercise, stress management, hydration, and sufficient rest, all of which are crucial for maintaining immune health. By combining these habits with a diet rich in healing foods like cayenne pepper, O'Neill's approach aims to foster a strong foundation for long-term health. Her belief is that boosting the immune system naturally can provide the body with the resources it needs to prevent illness and maintain optimal health, thereby reducing the reliance on pharmaceuticals and invasive medical interventions.

Brief on the Purpose of the Guide: Using Cayenne Pepper to Boost Immunity and Support Overall Wellness

The purpose of this guide is to provide readers with an in-depth look at the many ways cayenne pepper can be incorporated into daily life to promote immune health and overall wellness. While cayenne is often relegated to the kitchen as a spice, this guide aims to showcase its true potential as a healing powerhouse that can support and fortify the immune system. From dietary applications to topical uses and home remedies, this guide offers a comprehensive toolkit of practical recipes, treatments, and safety tips inspired by Barbara O'Neill's principles.

In today's fast-paced environment, numerous individuals encounter greater exposure to harmful microorganisms and elevated stress levels, which can adversely affect their immune systems. Rather than relying on regular antibiotic treatments and over-the-counter medications, a growing number of individuals are exploring natural and effective alternatives. Cayenne pepper, when incorporated into a holistic wellness regimen, serves as a potent ally in enhancing the body's innate ability to combat illnesses, infections, and inflammatory issues.

This guide is designed for those who seek to enhance their well-being through the use of natural, minimally processed ingredients that align with the body's innate healing abilities. Every chapter delves into a distinct facet of cayenne pepper's remarkable properties, highlighting its potential to enhance immunity and aid in detoxification, as well as its effectiveness in alleviating pain and promoting heart health. Additionally, the guide offers valuable information on the diverse uses of cayenne, encompassing healing recipes, invigorating tonics, soothing teas, topical salves, and beyond.

This guide is crafted for those navigating chronic health challenges or anyone aiming to enhance their immunity and overall vitality. It provides you with the essential insights to incorporate cayenne pepper into your wellness routine safely and effectively. By adhering to these principles, individuals can empower themselves regarding their health, enhance their immune systems, and adopt a lifestyle that emphasizes holistic well-being.

Ultimately, this guide transcends the focus on cayenne pepper; it emphasizes embracing a comprehensive lifestyle that honors the healing potential of nature's remedies. Highlighting the importance of equilibrium, restraint, and regularity, Barbara O'Neill's insights lead individuals to a profound comprehension of how to utilize the healing benefits of cayenne pepper in conjunction with various lifestyle habits for enduring wellness and vigor. By making small, practical changes in daily routines, this guide invites readers to begin a journey toward overall well-being, harnessing the versatile and restorative qualities of cayenne pepper.

CHAPTER 2

The Knowledge Behind Cayenne Pepper's Health Advantages

Cayenne's Anti-inflammatory and Antioxidant Benefits

The remarkable health advantages of cayenne pepper are primarily attributed to its strong anti-inflammatory and antioxidant characteristics, which enhance the body's capacity to handle inflammation and fight against oxidative stress. The main bioactive component in cayenne, capsaicin, is crucial for alleviating inflammation by suppressing the action of pro-inflammatory agents. Capsaicin operates at the cellular level to diminish the generation of inflammatory markers, including substance P—a neuropeptide linked to pain transmission and inflammatory reactions. By regulating these indicators, cayenne aids in alleviating inflammation-related issues such as arthritis, muscle discomfort, and joint pain.

Moreover, cayenne pepper boasts a wealth of antioxidants, such as vitamins A and C, which work to neutralize free radicals—those unstable molecules responsible for cellular damage and linked to aging and various diseases. These powerful compounds safeguard cells by counteracting free radicals, preventing potential harm to cellular DNA and proteins. Vitamin A plays a vital role in supporting immune cell function and maintaining skin integrity, which is essential for the body's primary defense against pathogens. Meanwhile, Vitamin C is recognized for its ability to stimulate immune cells and mitigate oxidative stress, making it indispensable for a robust immune system.

Chronic inflammation and oxidative stress are associated with numerous long-term health conditions, including heart disease, cancer, and autoimmune issues. By diminishing these inflammatory and oxidative processes, cayenne pepper serves as a protective agent against these conditions, fostering overall well-being and longevity. The properties of cayenne pepper, known for their anti-inflammatory and antioxidant effects, play a crucial role in boosting immune strength and reducing the likelihood of chronic health problems.
The Effects of Cayenne Pepper on Heart Health and Blood Flow

The influence of cayenne pepper on cardiovascular health is yet another domain where research underscores its impressive advantages. Cayenne enhances circulation by boosting blood flow and fortifying blood vessel walls, thereby ensuring that oxygen and vital nutrients are delivered efficiently to all parts of the body. This improved circulation aids in eliminating toxins and metabolic waste, lightening the burden on essential organs and promoting overall well-being. The warming properties of capsaicin enhance blood circulation, rendering cayenne especially advantageous for individuals experiencing cold extremities, sluggish blood flow, or cardiovascular concerns.

Consuming cayenne pepper regularly may help lower levels of "bad" LDL cholesterol and triglycerides, which are both contributors to clogged arteries and a heightened risk of heart disease. Capsaicin may also play a role in enhancing blood lipid profiles, which can aid in preventing plaque accumulation and decreasing the chances of cardiovascular incidents like heart attacks and strokes. By mitigating these risk factors, cayenne pepper supports healthier blood vessels and enhances the strength of the cardiovascular system.

Furthermore, cayenne pepper might assist in maintaining blood pressure levels. Research shows that capsaicin has the ability to expand blood vessels, which may enhance circulation and possibly reduce blood pressure levels. This effect is especially advantageous for those dealing with hypertension, given that elevated blood pressure poses a considerable risk for heart disease and stroke. Furthermore, the significant potassium levels found in cayenne contribute to cardiovascular wellness by assisting in the regulation of sodium levels within the body, thereby promoting effective blood pressure control.

The Benefits of Capsaicin for Alleviating Discomfort and Boosting Immune Health

Cayenne pepper is well-regarded for its scientifically backed ability to alleviate pain, largely attributed to the compound capsaicin. This compound is commonly found in topical pain relief creams and patches, functioning by reducing substance P levels in nerve cells. Substance P plays a crucial role in conveying pain signals to the brain; therefore, a reduction in its levels leads to a decrease in pain perception. Cayenne serves as a powerful natural solution for addressing different kinds of pain, such as joint discomfort from arthritis, nerve-related pain, and headaches.

Capsaicin offers gentle pain-relieving benefits, aiding in the alleviation of muscle soreness and tension when used on the skin. Studies indicate that the benefits of capsaicin for alleviating pain are cumulative, suggesting that consistent application over time may result in lasting decreases in pain sensitivity. For individuals experiencing chronic pain, cayenne pepper presents a natural option to pharmaceutical pain relievers, boasting fewer side effects and eliminating the risk of addiction.

Beyond alleviating discomfort, capsaicin significantly contributes to boosting the body's immune response. Cayenne enhances the body's innate defenses by stimulating the production of antibodies and immune cells. The anti-inflammatory properties of capsaicin play a crucial role in bolstering immunity, since ongoing inflammation can weaken immune function and increase vulnerability to infections. The immune-enhancing qualities of cayenne render it an essential ally in the fight against colds, flu, and various respiratory infections. Furthermore, capsaicin exhibits gentle antibacterial and antiviral characteristics, offering an extra measure of protection against harmful pathogens.

Advantages for Digestive Health, Metabolic Function, and Cleansing

The advantages of cayenne pepper for digestive health are thoroughly established. Capsaicin encourages the creation of digestive enzymes and gastric juices, vital for the breakdown of food and the absorption of nutrients. Cayenne supports the digestive process, aiding in the alleviation of symptoms such as indigestion, bloating, and gas. Furthermore, capsaicin has the ability to encourage peristalsis, promoting the rhythmic movement of muscles within the digestive system, which facilitates the seamless transit of food through the intestines and helps avert complications such as constipation.

The influence of cayenne on digestion significantly contributes to overall gut wellness, which is intricately linked to the body's immune capabilities. The gentle antibacterial qualities of pepper can assist in managing harmful gut bacteria, lowering the chances of infections and fostering a harmonious gut microbiome. A well-functioning gut is crucial for a strong immune system, with around 70% of immune cells found in the gastrointestinal tract. Incorporating cayenne pepper into your diet can significantly contribute to sustaining excellent gut health, thereby bolstering the body's natural immune defenses.

Cayenne pepper is well-known for its ability to enhance metabolism, which is why it is frequently included in weight management approaches. Capsaicin induces a thermogenic response, elevating the body's core temperature and promoting the burning of calories. Research indicates that capsaicin enhances metabolic rate and promotes fat oxidation, aiding the body in burning calories more effectively. Cayenne serves as an excellent resource for individuals looking to naturally boost their metabolism and control their weight effectively.

Moreover, cayenne pepper aids in the body's natural cleansing processes. The circulatory advantages improve the body's capacity to eliminate toxins via sweat and urine. Cayenne invigorates the lymphatic system, playing a crucial role in the collection and elimination of waste products and pathogens from the body's tissues. Cayenne plays a vital role in enhancing the lymphatic system, aiding the body in eliminating toxins that may otherwise overwhelm the immune system and contribute to chronic inflammation. Improved detoxification aids the liver, kidneys, and various organs that filter and remove toxins, leading to a purer internal environment.

Furthermore, the digestive and detoxifying qualities of cayenne play a significant role in supporting liver health. Capsaicin may offer protective benefits for liver cells against oxidative stress and inflammation, factors that can compromise liver function as time progresses. A well-functioning liver is crucial for effective detoxification, as it is key in processing and eliminating toxins from the blood. Cayenne pepper enhances liver function, which in turn fosters overall health, boosting energy levels and strengthening the body's defenses against illness.

The research surrounding cayenne pepper's health advantages uncovers a rich array of possibilities for improving wellness and warding off illness. The remarkable anti-inflammatory and antioxidant qualities contribute to lowering the risk of chronic diseases, while also enhancing circulation and promoting cardiovascular well-being, ultimately fortifying the heart and blood vessels. The distinctive properties of capsaicin in alleviating pain and enhancing immune function position cayenne as a multifaceted solution for pain management and bolstering the body's natural defenses. Ultimately, its advantages for digestion, metabolism, and detoxification offer essential support for sustaining optimal health, enabling cayenne pepper to function as a comprehensive, natural remedy.

CHAPTER 3

The Role of Cayenne Pepper in Supporting Immunity

How Cayenne Enhances Immune Function

Cayenne pepper significantly contributes to enhancing the immune system via various essential mechanisms. Central to its immune-boosting qualities is capsaicin, the active component that gives the pepper its heat and contributes to numerous health advantages. Capsaicin plays a role in bolstering the immune system by alleviating inflammation, a frequent root cause of various diseases and immune-related issues.

Alleviating Inflammation: Chronic inflammation has the potential to diminish the immune response, rendering the body more vulnerable to infections and diseases. Capsaicin is known to suppress the production of pro-inflammatory cytokines and mediators, leading to a decrease in inflammatory responses. By minimizing inflammation, the immune system can operate with greater efficiency, enhancing its ability to tackle potential threats like pathogens and toxins. Cayenne pepper plays a significant role in moderating inflammatory processes, thereby boosting the body's overall immune function and resilience.

Supporting the Body's Cleansing Processes: Detoxification plays a vital role in supporting the immune system, as it is essential for the body to efficiently remove toxins and waste products to achieve optimal health. Cayenne pepper enhances detoxification by invigorating the circulatory and lymphatic systems, crucial for the movement and removal of toxins. Enhanced circulation promotes the efficient elimination of waste from cells, while a well-functioning lymphatic system aids in the removal of pathogens and debris. By enhancing these detoxification processes, cayenne bolsters the immune system's capacity to combat infections and uphold harmony within the body.

Furthermore, the abundant vitamin C found in cayenne pepper enhances immune function by promoting the production of white blood cells, essential for combating infections. These vital cells play a crucial role in recognizing and eliminating harmful invaders, thereby strengthening the body's natural defenses. The antioxidants found in cayenne, including beta-carotene and flavonoids, serve to shield immune cells from oxidative stress, thereby ensuring their optimal performance as protectors against illness.

The Role of Cayenne Pepper in Combating Infections and Averting Illnesses

The capacity of cayenne pepper to boost immune function results in a strong shield against infections and ailments. Cayenne is particularly renowned for its ability to bolster the immune system, effectively combating common infections like colds and the flu. The warming effects encourage perspiration, aiding in the removal of toxins and pathogens from the body, while enhancing circulation allows immune cells to swiftly reach the impacted areas.

Studies show that capsaicin possesses antimicrobial properties, effectively targeting bacteria, fungi, and viruses. Cayenne pepper serves as a potent ally in the fight against infections. Research indicates that capsaicin possesses the ability to hinder the proliferation of specific bacteria linked to foodborne illnesses, including Salmonella and E. coli. Furthermore, cayenne is recognized for its antiviral qualities, which could potentially lessen both the intensity and length of viral infections, including the common cold.

Moreover, the beneficial effects of cayenne on digestion significantly contribute to enhancing immune health. A robust digestive system is intricately connected to a thriving immune system, with around 70% of immune cells found in the gut. Cayenne supports digestive health by enhancing the activity of digestive enzymes and fostering a thriving gut flora, thereby contributing to a balanced microbiome. A harmonious gut microbiome plays a crucial role in a robust immune response, as the presence of beneficial gut bacteria aids in educating the immune system to distinguish between harmful intruders and harmless elements.

Cayenne pepper may contribute to the prevention of chronic diseases that could weaken immune function. Health issues like obesity, diabetes, and heart disease can contribute to ongoing inflammation and hinder the immune system's capacity to effectively combat infections. Cayenne aids in enhancing metabolic health and encourages weight management through its thermogenic properties, thereby helping to reduce the risk of developing these conditions.

Moreover, cayenne contributes to enhancing cardiovascular health, ensuring optimal blood circulation and further aiding in the transport of immune cells throughout the body. This holistic perspective on wellness highlights the potency of cayenne pepper as a natural solution for boosting immunity and warding off illness.

Recommendations for Safe Usage and Suggested Dosages for Immune Support

Although cayenne pepper is typically safe for the majority, it is crucial to use it wisely to enhance its advantages for immune support and reduce any possible side effects. Here are some recommendations for safe usage and suggested dosages to boost immune health with cayenne pepper:

1. Varieties of Cayenne Pepper: - Cayenne pepper is available in multiple forms, such as fresh, dried, powdered, or as a extract. The powdered form is frequently utilized in culinary practices and can be effortlessly incorporated into soups, stews, or spice mixtures. Fresh cayenne peppers can enhance salads or smoothies with a delightful kick.

- Capsaicin supplements can be found on the market, yet it is wise to seek guidance from a healthcare professional prior to beginning any supplementation to ascertain the suitable dosage tailored to your specific requirements.

2. Suggested Amounts: - For overall immune enhancement, a daily intake of 1/4 to 1/2 teaspoon of cayenne powder is frequently advised. This can be effortlessly integrated into your culinary creations or drinks.
- When utilizing cayenne in a capsule form, the usual dosages fall between 30 mg and 120 mg of capsaicin daily. Once more, seeking guidance from a knowledgeable healthcare professional is essential to ascertain the right dosage tailored to personal health conditions and objectives.

3. Gradual Introduction: For those who are just beginning to explore cayenne pepper, it's advisable to commence with a modest quantity and slowly elevate the dosage as your body becomes accustomed. This method can assist in reducing any possible digestive unease or sensitivity to the heat of the pepper.

4. Potential Side Effects: - Although cayenne pepper is generally well-tolerated, certain individuals might

encounter digestive discomfort, including heartburn, nausea, or stomach upset, especially when taken in excessive amounts. Those experiencing gastrointestinal concerns, like irritable bowel syndrome (IBS) or acid reflux, ought to exercise caution and might need to restrict their consumption.
- Cayenne may have interactions with specific medications, including blood thinners and those prescribed for high blood pressure. Thus, it is essential to seek guidance from a qualified healthcare provider if you are taking any medications or have pre-existing health issues.

5. Incorporation into Diet: - There are various methods to seamlessly include cayenne pepper in your everyday meals. Incorporating a dash of cayenne into your soups, stews, stir-fries, or marinades not only elevates the taste but also offers various health advantages. Consider incorporating cayenne into your smoothies, infusing it into salad dressings, or dusting it over popcorn for a delightful spicy treat.
- Crafting a cayenne-infused honey is a favored approach to seamlessly integrate cayenne into your dietary routine. Mix raw honey with cayenne pepper and allow it to steep for several days. This blend can be consumed by the spoonful

to enhance immune wellness or incorporated into tea for a calming drink.

6. Precautions: - It is advisable for pregnant and breastfeeding women to seek guidance from their healthcare provider prior to consuming substantial amounts of cayenne pepper, as elevated doses may not be recommended during these times.
- If you are aware of an allergy to chili peppers or have a history of severe reactions to spicy foods, it would be wise to avoid cayenne.

By adhering to these recommendations and integrating cayenne pepper into a well-rounded diet, one can effectively tap into its immune-enhancing benefits. Incorporating cayenne pepper into your routine can significantly boost your immune system and promote overall well-being, making it an invaluable component of a health-focused lifestyle.

Cayenne pepper provides a comprehensive strategy for bolstering the immune system, functioning through various processes like diminishing inflammation, facilitating detoxification, and combating infections. Cayenne pepper, with its remarkable health benefits, is a noteworthy natural remedy for boosting immunity and supporting overall wellness. By recognizing its benefits and following safe usage practices, individuals can incorporate cayenne pepper into their health regimen, strengthening their body's natural defenses against illness and disease.

CHAPTER 4

Healing Recipes with Cayenne Pepper

Cayenne pepper serves as a potent spice and a multifaceted ingredient, capable of elevating both the taste and health advantages of numerous dishes and beverages. This chapter delves into an array of restorative recipes that highlight the benefits of cayenne pepper, each crafted to enhance immunity and promote holistic well-being. From tonics and elixirs to smoothies, soups, and salads, these recipes beautifully blend the health benefits of cayenne with delightful flavors and simple preparation methods.

Potions and Remedies

Cayenne and Lemon Tonic for Immune Support

Components:
- 1 teaspoon cayenne pepper (either in powdered form or fresh)
- Juice from one lemon
- 1 tablespoon of unprocessed honey (optional)
- 2 cups of warm water
- A dash of sea salt (optional)

Guidelines:
1. In a glass or bowl, blend the cayenne pepper with the lemon juice.
2. Gradually incorporate the warm water, stirring gently until the cayenne is thoroughly blended.
3. For those who wish, incorporate honey to enhance sweetness and a dash of sea salt to elevate the flavor profile.
4. Mix well and consume while warm to fully experience the benefits.

Wellness Advantages:
This tonic utilizes the remarkable benefits of cayenne pepper, celebrated for its anti-inflammatory and immune-enhancing qualities. The vitamin C found in lemon serves to bolster immune function, while honey contributes its own antimicrobial properties and soothing effects. Regular consumption of this tonic can enhance your immune system, especially during the cold and flu season.

Cayenne Ginger Purifying Tonic

Components:
- 1 teaspoon of cayenne pepper - 1 tablespoon of freshly grated ginger - Juice from 1 lime
- 1 tablespoon of unprocessed honey (optional)
- 2 cups of water

Guidelines:
1. In a modest saucepan, allow the water to reach a gentle simmer.
2. Incorporate the grated ginger and cayenne pepper, allowing it to gently simmer for approximately 10 minutes.
3. Take it off the heat and allow it to cool a bit.
4. Carefully strain the mixture into a glass, ensuring to discard the ginger solids.
5. Incorporate the lime juice and honey, mixing thoroughly until well blended.
6. Savor it warm or chilled.

Wellness Advantages:
This detox elixir harmoniously blends the digestive advantages of ginger with the invigorating properties of cayenne. This combination enhances circulation and supports detoxification, making this beverage ideal for purifying the body. The addition of lime juice introduces a delightful zest while increasing vitamin C levels, thereby amplifying its beneficial effects on immune health.

Nourishing Blends and Infusions

Zesty Immunity Boosting Smoothie with Cayenne, Turmeric, and Ginger

Components:

- 1 cup of vibrant spinach or nutrient-rich kale
- 1 banana (either fresh or frozen)
- 1/2 cup chunks of pineapple or mango
- 1/2 teaspoon of cayenne pepper - 1/2 teaspoon of turmeric powder
- 1 tablespoon freshly grated ginger - 1 cup of coconut water or almond milk
- Optional ice cubes

Guidelines:
1. In a blender, mix together the spinach or kale, banana, pineapple or mango, cayenne pepper, turmeric powder, ginger, and either coconut water or almond milk.
2. Combine thoroughly until a silky consistency is achieved, incorporating ice cubes if you prefer a refreshing chill.
3. Sample the flavor and modify the sweetness as needed.

Wellness Advantages:
This lively smoothie is a treasure trove of nutrients, blending the soothing properties of cayenne, turmeric, and ginger with the rich vitamins and minerals present in fruits and greens. Spinach and kale are rich in antioxidants, while cayenne and ginger enhance the flavor and stimulate metabolism. This smoothie enhances immune health while delivering a boost of energy and hydration.

Infusion of Herbal Tea with Cayenne for Relief from Cold and Flu

Components:
- 1 cup of hot water - 1 teaspoon of cayenne pepper - 1 teaspoon of dried thyme or 1 sprig of fresh thyme - 1 teaspoon of honey (optional)
- Juice from half a lemon

Guidelines:
1. Infuse the thyme in hot water for approximately 5 minutes.
2. Incorporate the cayenne pepper and mix thoroughly.
3. Strain out the thyme and incorporate honey and lemon juice according to your preference.
4. Enjoy it warm to fully embrace its benefits.

Wellness Advantages:
This infusion of herbal tea melds the warming essence of cayenne with the antimicrobial benefits of thyme, complemented by the calming attributes of honey and lemon. This remedy aids in alleviating cold symptoms by clearing nasal passages and calming sore throats, with the added benefit of cayenne boosting circulation and supporting the immune system.

Broths and Hearty Dishes

Cayenne-Infused Vegetable Broth for Soothing Inflammation

Components:
- 8 cups of water
- 2 carrots, finely chopped
- 2 chopped stalks of celery
- 1 onion, finely chopped
- 2 cloves of garlic, finely minced
- 1 teaspoon of cayenne pepper - 1 teaspoon of dried oregano
- 1 bay leaf
- Season with salt and pepper according to your preference

Guidelines:
1. In a spacious pot, combine water, carrots, celery, onion, garlic, cayenne pepper, oregano, and bay leaf.
2. Heat until boiling, then lower the temperature and let it gently simmer for 30-40 minutes.
3. Strain the broth to eliminate the vegetables, or blend them for a more robust texture.
4. Enhance the flavor with a sprinkle of salt and pepper to your preference before serving.

Wellness Advantages:
This cayenne-infused vegetable broth offers a delightful warmth while being abundant in vitamins and minerals

sourced from the vegetables. The anti-inflammatory qualities of cayenne enhance the nutrient-dense broth, rendering it a superb option for alleviating inflammation and promoting overall well-being.

Nourishing Chicken Broth Enhanced with Spicy Cayenne and Botanical Infusions

Components:
- 1 whole bird or 4 thigh portions
- 8 cups of chicken broth or water
- 2 carrots, finely sliced
- 2 celery stalks, finely sliced
- 1 onion, finely chopped
- 3 cloves of garlic, finely minced
- 1 teaspoon of cayenne pepper - 1 teaspoon of dried thyme - 1 teaspoon of dried rosemary
- Season with salt and pepper according to your preference - Use fresh parsley as a garnish

Guidelines:
1. In a spacious pot, place the chicken and immerse it in chicken broth or water.
2. Heat until boiling, then lower the heat and let it gently simmer for approximately 30 minutes or until the chicken is thoroughly cooked.
3. Take out the chicken and shred it, then place the meat back into the pot.

4. Incorporate carrots, celery, onion, garlic, cayenne pepper, thyme, and rosemary into the pot.
5. Allow it to simmer for another 20-30 minutes, adjusting the seasoning with salt and pepper according to your preference.
6. Present while warm, adorned with vibrant fresh parsley.

Wellness Advantages:
This nourishing chicken soup melds the comforting essence of a classic recipe with the enhanced wellness properties of cayenne and various herbs. Cayenne pepper enhances circulation and combats inflammation, while the nutrients found in chicken and vegetables offer vital support for recovery from illness.

Greens and Vinaigrettes

Zesty Cayenne Lemon Dressing for Immune Wellness

Components:
- 1/4 cup of olive oil - Juice from 1 lemon
- 1 teaspoon of cayenne pepper - 1 teaspoon of Dijon mustard - 1 clove of minced garlic
- Season with salt and pepper according to your preference

Guidelines:

1. In a small bowl or jar, blend together olive oil, lemon juice, cayenne pepper, Dijon mustard, and minced garlic.
2. Blend thoroughly by whisking or shaking until the mixture is harmonious.
3. Enhance the flavor with a pinch of salt and a dash of pepper according to your preference.

Wellness Advantages:
This vibrant dressing infuses a lively zest into any salad, while delivering immune-enhancing properties from the cayenne and lemon. This dressing combines the wholesome benefits of olive oil, which provides healthy fats essential for overall well-being, with the immune-enhancing qualities of garlic. It's a superb option for elevating nutrient-dense salads.

Avocado and Cayenne Immunity Salad

Components:
- 2 ripe avocados, diced - 1 cup cherry tomatoes, halved - 1/2 red onion, thinly sliced - 1 cucumber, diced
- 1 teaspoon of cayenne pepper - Juice from 1 lime
- Season with salt and pepper according to your preference - Garnish with fresh cilantro

Guidelines:

1. In a spacious bowl, blend together diced avocados, cherry tomatoes, finely chopped red onion, and refreshing cucumber.
2. In a distinct small bowl, combine cayenne pepper, lime juice, salt, and pepper.
3. Drizzle the dressing over the salad and softly mix to blend the flavors.
4. Enhance the dish with a sprinkle of fresh cilantro just before serving.

Wellness Advantages:
This invigorating avocado salad is brimming with nourishing fats, essential vitamins, and minerals, while the addition of cayenne provides a zesty flair and boosts immune health. The blend of fresh vegetables offers a wealth of antioxidants that help counter oxidative stress, elevating this salad to a wholesome enhancement for your meals.

Adding cayenne pepper to your daily meals can be a delightful and tasty method to enhance immunity and support overall well-being. These recipes serve as a foundation, encouraging you to delve into the world of cayenne and discover its remarkable properties as a healing element. Cayenne pepper, whether incorporated into tonics, smoothies, soups, or salads, provides a wealth of health advantages while delighting your palate.

CHAPTER 5

Cayenne Solutions for Everyday Health Concerns

Cayenne pepper serves as a delightful spice while also acting as a powerful solution for a range of health concerns. The active component, capsaicin, is recognized for its healing properties, rendering cayenne a potent natural remedy for various conditions, including colds, digestive troubles, pain, and skin issues. This chapter delves into the ways cayenne can be harnessed to address prevalent health issues and promote overall wellness, offering recipes and remedies for integration into your everyday routine.

Natural Remedies for Cold and Flu

The warming qualities of cayenne pepper, along with its ability to enhance immune function, render it a superb solution for alleviating cold and flu symptoms. Here are various cayenne remedies to assist in alleviating congestion, sore throats, and other associated issues:

Cayenne and Honey Gargle for Throat Discomfort

Components:
- 1 cup of warm water - 1 teaspoon of cayenne pepper - 1 tablespoon of honey

Guidelines:
1. Combine the cayenne pepper and honey in warm water, stirring until completely dissolved.
2. Swish the blend in your mouth for 30 seconds before expelling it. Reapply as necessary.

Wellness Advantages:
This calming gargle harnesses the natural pain-relieving qualities of cayenne to ease throat discomfort, while honey provides antimicrobial benefits and helps to soothe irritation.

Steam Inhalation with Cayenne Pepper for Sinus Congestion

Components:
- 1 teaspoon of cayenne pepper - 4 cups of boiling water - A towel

Guidelines:
1. In a spacious bowl, combine the boiling water with cayenne pepper.
2. Bend over the bowl, ensuring to drape a towel over your head to capture the steam effectively.

3. Breathe in the steam for 5-10 minutes, ensuring you maintain a safe distance to prevent any burns.

Wellness Advantages:
Inhaling steam infused with cayenne can effectively open nasal passages, alleviate congestion, and enhance breathing. Capsaicin may assist in thinning mucus, facilitating easier expulsion.

Support for Digestion

Cayenne pepper is known to enhance digestion and provide relief from common gastrointestinal discomforts like indigestion, bloating, and gas. Here are some natural solutions and formulations for promoting digestive wellness:

Cayenne Ginger Infusion for Digestive Relief

Components:
- 1 teaspoon of cayenne pepper - 1 tablespoon of freshly grated ginger - 1 tablespoon of honey (optional) - 2 cups of water

Guidelines:
1. In a saucepan, bring water to a boil and incorporate ginger and cayenne.

2. Allow it to gently simmer for approximately 10 minutes, then carefully strain it into a cup.
3. Incorporate honey if you wish, and enjoy it warm.

Wellness Advantages:
This tea merges the digestive advantages of ginger with the stimulating properties of cayenne, enhancing overall digestion and easing discomfort associated with indigestion.

Cayenne Detox Tonic for Digestive Relief

Components:
- 1 tablespoon of apple cider vinegar - 1 teaspoon of cayenne pepper - 1 tablespoon of honey (optional) - 1 cup of water

Guidelines:
1. In a glass, blend all the components and mix thoroughly until they are harmoniously combined.
2. Consume it prior to meals to support digestion and alleviate bloating.

Wellness Advantages:
This detox tonic harnesses the digestive properties of apple cider vinegar and cayenne to support gut health, alleviate bloating, and enhance digestion.

Natural Approaches to Pain and Inflammation Relief

Cayenne pepper is celebrated for its pain-relieving and inflammation-reducing qualities, proving beneficial for alleviating discomfort and swelling linked to arthritis, joint pain, and muscle soreness. Here are a few natural solutions to explore:

Cayenne Pepper Soothing Balm

Components:
- 1/2 cup coconut oil - 2 tablespoons cayenne pepper - 1 tablespoon beeswax (optional, for a thicker consistency)

Guidelines:
1. Gently combine the coconut oil and beeswax (if incorporating) in a double boiler until fully melted.
2. Gently incorporate the cayenne pepper until it is uniformly blended.
3. Let the blend cool and solidify, then carefully place it into a glass jar.

Wellness Advantages:
Utilizing this cream on aching joints and muscles may offer soothing relief from discomfort and swelling. Capsaicin functions by inhibiting pain signals, providing a natural approach to pain relief free from the adverse effects

associated with pharmaceutical alternatives.

Cayenne and Turmeric Soothing Smoothie

Components:
- 1/2 teaspoon of cayenne pepper - 1 teaspoon of turmeric powder
- 1 cup of almond milk or coconut water
- 1 ripe banana
- 1 tablespoon of almond butter (optional)

Guidelines:
1. Combine all the components thoroughly until you achieve a smooth consistency.
2. Transfer into a glass and savor right away.

Wellness Advantages:
This smoothie blends the soothing qualities of cayenne and turmeric, offering a delightful and nourishing method to support the body's natural response to inflammation.

Dermal Wellness

Cayenne pepper offers advantages beyond internal wellness; it can also enhance the condition of the skin. The ability to enhance circulation and its abundance of nutrients contribute to its effectiveness in addressing acne, rejuvenating the skin, and minimizing the appearance of aging signs. Discover these cayenne-infused solutions for enhancing skin vitality:

Cayenne and Honey Facial Treatment for Blemishes

Components:
- 1 teaspoon of cayenne pepper - 2 tablespoons of honey - 1 teaspoon of lemon juice

Guidelines:
1. Combine all the components to create a smooth paste.
2. Gently apply to the affected areas, steering clear of the delicate skin around the eyes.
Allow it to sit for 10-15 minutes, then gently rinse with warm water.

Wellness Advantages:
This face mask utilizes the antibacterial benefits of cayenne to combat acne, while honey contributes moisture and promotes healing. This mask may assist in alleviating inflammation and fostering a clearer complexion.

Cayenne Invigorating Body Exfoliant

Components:

- 1/2 cup of natural sweetener or mineral-rich salt
- 1/4 cup of coconut oil - 1 teaspoon of cayenne pepper

Guidelines:
1. Blend all components in a bowl to create a scrub.
2. Delicately apply to damp skin while in the shower, paying special attention to areas that require rejuvenation.
3. Rinse thoroughly and then apply your moisturizer.

Wellness Advantages:
This scrub gently sloughs away dead skin cells while enhancing circulation, resulting in a refreshed and revitalized appearance for your skin. The cayenne pepper promotes circulation, potentially improving the skin's overall look.
Cayenne Youth Renewal Elixir

Components:
- 2 tablespoons of a base oil, such as jojoba or sweet almond oil
- 1 teaspoon of cayenne pepper - 1 teaspoon of vitamin E oil

Guidelines:
1. Combine all components in a small glass vessel.
2. Gently massage a few drops onto the face and neck.

Wellness Advantages:
This serum is designed to enhance skin elasticity and diminish the visibility of fine lines. The invigorating properties of cayenne enhance circulation, contributing to a vibrant, youthful complexion, while vitamin E oil provides essential nourishment and protection for the skin.

Cayenne pepper stands out as an exceptional natural solution, capable of addressing a variety of everyday health challenges, including colds, digestive troubles, pain, and skin issues. Incorporating cayenne into your daily regimen with these remedies and recipes allows you to tap into its powerful healing benefits for your overall well-being. Whether taken in tonics, used in creams, or incorporated into beauty treatments, cayenne pepper provides an array of advantages that enhance well-being and vigor.

CHAPTER 6

Utilizing Cayenne Topically for Alleviating Discomfort

Cayenne pepper, celebrated for its spiciness and taste, also boasts powerful analgesic and anti-inflammatory qualities, rendering it a valuable natural solution for alleviating pain. The active compound found in cayenne, capsaicin, is known for its ability to relieve pain associated with various conditions, such as arthritis, muscle soreness, and neuropathic pain. This chapter delves into the art of crafting homemade cayenne salves and rubs, presenting a detailed step-by-step guide for preparing capsaicin cream, along with vital safety tips for its topical use.

Crafting Your Own Cayenne Pepper Salves and Rubs

Crafting your own cayenne salves and rubs is a straightforward process that can yield powerful relief from pain and inflammation. The method generally entails steeping cayenne pepper in a carrier oil, which can subsequently be blended with additional calming components to formulate a powerful topical solution.

Fundamental Cayenne Infused Oil

Components:
- 1 cup olive oil (or any preferred carrier oil)
- 2 tablespoons of dried cayenne pepper
- Optional: 1 tablespoon of beeswax (to achieve a more substantial consistency in your salve)

Instructions: 1. Craft the Herbal Infusion:
- In a small saucepan, gently blend the olive oil and cayenne pepper over low heat. - Let the blend infuse gently for approximately 30-60 minutes, stirring from time to time. Exercise care to avoid boiling, as excessive heat can diminish the valuable qualities of the oil and cayenne.

2. Strain the Oil: - Once the infusion period has concluded, take the saucepan off the heat.
- Employ a fine mesh strainer or cheesecloth to carefully filter out the cayenne pepper, allowing only the infused oil to remain.

3. Cool and Store: - Allow the oil to reach room temperature, then carefully pour it into a clean, dark glass bottle or jar for optimal preservation. Keep it in a cool, dark environment to maintain its effectiveness.

4. Optional: Create a Healing Salve: - For a richer texture, gently melt beeswax using a double boiler and blend it with the cayenne-infused oil until thoroughly integrated. Transfer the blend into suitable containers and allow it to cool and solidify naturally.

Health Benefits: This cayenne-infused oil serves as an excellent foundation for pain relief salves, can be incorporated into lotions, or applied directly to alleviate discomfort in sore muscles and joints.

Procedure for Crafting a Capsaicin Cream to Alleviate Joint and Muscle Discomfort

Capsaicin cream serves as a potent solution for joint and muscle pain, aiding in the reduction of inflammation and providing relief from discomfort. Here's a simple approach to crafting your own capsaicin cream:

DIY Capsaicin Ointment

Components:
- 1/4 cup oil infused with cayenne (prepared as previously outlined)
- 1/4 cup of coconut oil (or shea butter for a richer consistency)
- 1/4 cup beeswax (for enhancing consistency)

- Optional: 10-20 drops of essential oils (like eucalyptus or peppermint for enhanced relief and a pleasant aroma)

Instructions: 1. Melt the Base: - In a double boiler, blend the cayenne-infused oil, coconut oil, and beeswax together. Warm slowly until all ingredients are fully melted and harmoniously blended. Gently stir from time to time to promote a harmonious blend.

2. Incorporate Essential Oils: - After melting, take the mixture off the heat. Should you choose to include them, blend in your selected essential oils and mix thoroughly to ensure a harmonious integration.

3. Cool and Store: - Carefully transfer the warm blend into small jars or containers. Let it rest at room temperature until it fully solidifies. Keep the cream in a cool, dark environment for optimal preservation.

4. Application: - For optimal results, take a small quantity of the cream and delicately massage it into the affected area of the skin. Begin with a modest amount to evaluate how your skin responds before increasing the application.

Health Benefits: The blend of cayenne and coconut oil in this cream offers effective pain relief while also delivering nourishing moisture to the skin.

Guidelines for Safe Application on Skin

Although cayenne pepper and its derivatives can provide notable pain relief, adhering to safety guidelines is crucial for effective and safe application. Here are some essential safety guidelines to consider:

1. Perform a Patch Test: - Prior to using any cayenne-infused product on a broader area, it is advisable to conduct a patch test on a small section of skin (such as the inner forearm). Allow a full day to observe for any negative responses, including redness, itching, or a burning sensation.

2. Begin with Minimal Quantities: - When incorporating cayenne products into your routine for the first time, it's wise to start with a small amount to gauge your tolerance. If the feeling becomes overwhelming or bothersome, cleanse the area with soap and water right away. 3. Steer Clear of Delicate Regions: - Refrain from using cayenne-infused products on delicate areas, such as the face, around the eyes, or on

compromised skin. These regions are particularly susceptible to discomfort and negative responses.

4. Cleanse Hands Post-Application: - Following the application of cayenne products, ensure you cleanse your hands thoroughly to prevent any accidental transfer of capsaicin to your eyes or mucous membranes.

5. Think About Dilution: - When utilizing cayenne pepper directly (such as in a DIY salve), it's wise to dilute it with a carrier oil or other calming components to minimize the chance of irritation.

6. Seek Guidance from a Specialist: - If you have any existing skin conditions or are pregnant or nursing, it is advisable to seek guidance from a specialist before incorporating cayenne pepper products for pain relief.

Optimal Approaches for Managing Skin Sensitivity

Skin sensitivity differs among individuals, and knowing how to properly care for your skin when incorporating cayenne is essential for a beneficial experience. Here are some optimal approaches:

1. Moisturize Regularly: - After using cayenne-infused creams, it's essential to apply a calming moisturizer to nourish and safeguard the skin. Seek out botanical elements such as aloe vera or shea butter to reduce discomfort.

2. Observe Skin Response: - Take note of how your skin reacts following the application of cayenne products. Should you observe ongoing redness, discomfort, or irritation, it is advisable to cease use and seek the guidance of a dermatologist.

3. Minimize Sun Exposure: - Following the application of cayenne-infused products, steer clear of direct sunlight on the treated area. Capsaicin has the potential to heighten skin sensitivity, rendering it more susceptible to sunburn.

4. Reflect on Usage Regularity: - Reduce the frequency of use to prevent overloading the skin. Begin with one or two applications each day, and modify as necessary according to your personal tolerance and requirements.

5. Tailored Blends: - Explore blends that incorporate calming elements like calendula oil, chamomile, or lavender to elevate the soothing properties of your cayenne-infused creations.

Cayenne pepper serves as a multifaceted and potent natural solution for alleviating pain. By crafting your own salves and rubs, you can tap into its therapeutic qualities to effectively alleviate pain and reduce inflammation. Choosing cayenne-infused oils, creams, or straightforward topical applications can offer considerable relief for discomfort in joints and muscles. It is essential to adhere to safety guidelines and best practices to guarantee a beneficial experience when applying cayenne for topical pain relief. With the proper method, cayenne pepper can transform into a beneficial element in your holistic health repertoire.

CHAPTER 7

The Role of Cayenne Pepper in Detoxification and Weight Management

Cayenne pepper transcends its role as a mere spice that enhances the heat of your meals; it serves as a formidable partner in the journey of detoxification and weight management. Cayenne pepper, abundant in capsaicin, may aid in enhancing the body's natural detox processes, boost metabolism, and contribute to effective weight management. This chapter delves into the ways cayenne aids in detoxification, shares recipes for detox beverages and body cleanses, and presents suggestions for integrating cayenne into your weight loss plan.

The Role of Cayenne in Enhancing Detoxification Processes

The process of detoxification involves the body's natural ability to remove toxins and harmful substances. Cayenne pepper supports this process in multiple ways:

1. Enhancing Circulation: - Capsaicin promotes improved blood flow, facilitating the transport of oxygen and

nutrients to cells while assisting in the elimination of waste products. Enhanced blood flow aids the liver and kidneys, essential organs that play a crucial role in the detoxification process.

2. Boosting Digestive Health: - Cayenne pepper encourages the secretion of essential digestive fluids, such as saliva, gastric juices, and bile. This aids in the breakdown of food and enhances nutrient absorption, while also encouraging the removal of waste.

3. Nurturing the Liver: - The liver serves as the body's main detoxification organ, and cayenne may offer protection against oxidative stress thanks to its antioxidant qualities. It could potentially support liver function, aiding in the breakdown of toxins.

4. Encouraging Perspiration: - The thermogenic properties of cayenne stimulate an increase in body temperature, encouraging perspiration. Sweating serves as a natural means of detoxification, enabling the body to release impurities through the skin.

5. Balancing Properties: - Despite its spiciness, cayenne contributes to an alkalizing effect on the body following digestion. This equilibrium aids in

counteracting acidity, which may be advantageous for diminishing inflammation and promoting overall well-being.

Formulations for Cayenne Detox Beverages and Bodily Purifications

Adding cayenne to detox beverages and cleansing routines can significantly boost their efficacy. Discover these delightful and straightforward recipes that harness the cleansing properties of cayenne pepper:

1. Zesty Lemon Cleanse Beverage

Components:
- 1 cup of warm water - Juice from 1 fresh lemon
- 1/4 teaspoon of cayenne pepper - 1 tablespoon of raw honey (optional)

Guidelines:
1. Combine warm water with freshly squeezed lemon juice in a glass.
2. Incorporate cayenne pepper and mix thoroughly until fully blended.
3. If you wish, incorporate honey to enhance the sweetness.
4. Consume this cleansing drink first thing in the morning on an empty stomach.

Health Benefits: This beverage invigorates metabolism, enhances liver function, and delivers a rich source of vitamin C.

2. Detox Tonic with Cayenne and Apple Cider Vinegar

Components:
- 1 tablespoon of apple cider vinegar - 1/4 teaspoon of cayenne pepper - 1 cup of water
- Juice from half a lime or lemon
- Optional: a dash of sea salt
Guidelines:
1. In a glass, combine the apple cider vinegar with cayenne pepper.
2. Incorporate water along with lime or lemon juice, mixing thoroughly until everything is harmoniously blended.
3. Consume this tonic each day to enhance digestion and promote detoxification.

Health Benefits: This tonic merges the cleansing properties of cayenne with apple cider vinegar, recognized for its potential to harmonize pH levels and enhance digestive wellness.

3. Spicy Detox Smoothie with Cayenne Pepper

Components:

- 1 banana
- 1 cup of nutrient-rich spinach or kale
- 1/2 cup of pure almond milk, free from added sugars
- 1/4 teaspoon of cayenne pepper - 1 tablespoon of chia seeds (optional)
- Optional ice cubes

Guidelines:
1. In a blender, blend together all the ingredients.
2. Combine thoroughly until you achieve a smooth and creamy consistency.
3. Transfer into a glass and savor the experience!

Health Benefits: This nutrient-rich smoothie offers a blend of fiber, vitamins, and minerals, with cayenne boosting metabolism and supporting detoxification.

Guidelines for Incorporating Cayenne to Enhance Metabolism and Aid Weight Management

Integrating cayenne pepper into your everyday regimen may aid in weight loss and enhance metabolic function. Here are some insightful suggestions for utilizing cayenne to its fullest potential:

1. Begin Gradually: - For those unfamiliar with cayenne pepper, it's wise to introduce it in modest quantities to

gauge your body's response. Slowly enhance the amount as your body acclimates to its warmth.

2. Integrate into Dishes: - Enhance your dishes by sprinkling cayenne pepper on salads, soups, stews, or roasted vegetables. This not only elevates taste but also offers advantages for metabolism.

3. Establish a Cayenne Detox Protocol: - It may be beneficial to designate particular days for cleansing your system. Integrate cayenne-infused beverages and dishes into your regimen on these days to enhance your body's natural detoxification efforts.

4. Maintain Adequate Hydration: - Consuming ample amounts of water daily is crucial for the body's natural cleansing processes. Cayenne may elevate your thirst levels, so pay attention to your body's signals and maintain proper hydration.

5. Integrate with Additional Weight Management Tools: - To achieve optimal results, consider blending cayenne with additional natural weight loss support like green tea, ginger, or lemon. These components can harmonize to enhance metabolic function and support the process of fat reduction.

6. Be Conscious of Your Portions: - Although cayenne pepper may enhance metabolism, it is important to recognize that it is not a miraculous remedy for weight loss. Embrace a wholesome diet, be mindful of portion sizes, and engage in regular physical activity to achieve optimal outcomes.

7. Observe How Your Body Reacts: - Observe the responses of your body to cayenne pepper. If you encounter any discomfort or digestive concerns, consider modifying your intake or seek guidance from a qualified health practitioner.

8. Utilize as a Snack: - Think about preparing zesty snacks such as nuts seasoned with cayenne or flavorful popcorn. These can fulfill cravings while delivering the advantages of cayenne without an overload of calories.

Cayenne pepper is an excellent ally in the journey of detoxification and weight loss. By aiding the body's inherent detoxification processes, boosting metabolism, and offering delightful and nourishing recipes, cayenne can be effortlessly incorporated into your everyday life. Embrace the warmth of cayenne pepper, and discover its ability to enhance overall health, support detoxification, and aid in effective weight management. With a thoughtful perspective and the appropriate formulations, cayenne can serve as a powerful companion in your pursuit of improved well-being.

THE END

www.ingramcontent.com/pod-product-compliance
Lightning Source LLC
Chambersburg PA
CBHW070439290526
45791CB00005B/2037

* 9 7 8 1 3 0 0 8 9 1 5 9 8 *